I0490774

LIVING NATURALLY

A Comprehensive Introduction to Naturopathy

Philipp Frühwirth

CONTENTS

INTRODUCTION TO NATUROPATHY

Naturopathy is a holistic approach to healthcare that focuses on embracing the body's natural self-healing abilities. It is based on the principle that the body has an innate ability to heal itself, and treatments are directed towards supporting and promoting this ability. Unlike conventional medicine, which tends to rely heavily on drugs and surgery to treat illness, naturopathy is focused on preventive measures, education, and natural therapies.

One of the key goals of naturopathic medicine is to treat the whole person rather than just a particular condition or disease. Naturopaths use a variety of modalities such as homeopathy, acupuncture, herbal medicine, nutrition, and lifestyle modifications to address the root cause of the illness. This approach is known as "individualized medicine" and is based on the understanding that each person's unique circumstances must be taken into consideration in the treatment process.

Naturopathic medicine is not just about treating illness, but it is also about living a healthy and fulfilling life. It focuses on the importance of maintaining optimal health by adopting healthy lifestyle habits such as exercise, a balanced diet, and stress management techniques. By doing so, individuals can reduce their risk of developing chronic diseases and support their body's natural ability to heal itself.

The philosophy of naturopathy is based on six guiding principles:

1. The healing power of nature: Naturopathic medicine believes that the body has an innate ability to heal itself, and treatments

should focus on supporting this ability.

2. Identify and treat the root cause: Rather than just treating the symptoms of an illness, naturopaths focus on identifying and treating the underlying cause of the health issue.

3. Do no harm: Naturopaths use therapies that are safe and non-invasive, with the goal of minimizing the risk of harm or side effects.

4. Treat the whole person: Naturopaths view the body as a whole, taking into consideration all aspects of a person's health and lifestyle habits.

5. Prevention is key: Naturopathy places significant emphasis on preventative medicine and maintaining optimal health.

6. Education is essential: Naturopaths believe that educating individuals about their health and providing them with the tools they need to maintain optimal health is key to long-term health and wellness.

In conclusion, naturopathy provides a holistic approach to healthcare by empowering individuals to take control of their health and well-being. It embraces the body's natural healing ability and uses a variety of natural therapies and lifestyle modifications to support optimal health. By incorporating naturopathic principles into our lives, we can take steps towards living a healthier and more fulfilling life.

NATUROPATHIC PHILOSOPHY AND PRINCIPLES

Naturopathy is a system of medicine that is based on natural healing and approach towards treating diseases. Naturopathy focuses on the body's innate ability to heal itself, and its principles are based on the belief that there is a vital force within the body that regulates the overall health.

The philosophy of naturopathy is based on treating the root cause of disease, rather than just the symptoms. The goal of naturopathic medicine is to promote health and prevent disease, rather than just treating the symptoms of an illness. Naturopathy is rooted in the belief that the body has the ability to heal itself, and that the role of the naturopath is to facilitate that process by identifying and removing barriers to health.

Naturopathic medicine is founded on six principles that make up the basis of this approach to healing. These principles are:

1. First, Do No Harm: This principle stresses the importance of using the least invasive and least harmful treatments to treat an illness.

2. The Healing Power of Nature: The body has an innate ability to heal itself, and Naturopathy works to support this process through natural remedies and treatments.

3. Identify and Treat the Root Cause: Naturopathy seeks to identify and treat the underlying cause of the illness, rather than just treating the symptoms.

4. Treat the Whole Person: Naturopathy takes into account the physical, emotional, mental, social, and spiritual aspects of

a person to provide a treatment that encompasses the whole person.

5. Prevention: Naturopathy seeks to prevent illness by promoting health and wellness through lifestyle changes, natural remedies, and other preventative measures.

6. Doctor as Teacher: Naturopathy emphasizes educating the patient about their health and providing them with the tools and knowledge they need to maintain optimal health.

The philosophy of naturopathy is based on the idea that the body is constantly striving for optimum health, and that our role as naturopaths is to provide support and guidance to facilitate this process. By treating the whole person and working to remove barriers to health, naturopathic medicine helps patients achieve long-lasting wellness and vitality.

HISTORY OF NATUROPATHY

Naturopathy is a holistic healthcare approach that emphasizes natural and non-invasive techniques for the treatment of disease and promotion of optimal health. The practice of naturopathy dates back thousands of years to ancient healing practices in India, China, and Greece.

The principles of naturopathy were first formulated in the late 19th century by German physician Benedict Lust. Lust had personally experienced the healing powers of natural remedies and was inspired to share these methods with others. He coined the term "naturopathy" to describe a system of medicine that emphasizes the body's natural healing powers and the use of natural therapies to support these processes.

In the early 20th century, Lust brought naturopathy to the United States and founded the first naturopathic college. Over time, other schools were founded and the practice of naturopathy began to gain acceptance in the United States and other parts of the world.

Throughout the 20th century, naturopathy underwent some changes and further developments. The practice became more standardized and regulated as more countries and states established laws and regulations for licensing naturopathic practitioners.

In the present day, naturopathy is an established healthcare profession that is recognized in many countries around the world. Naturopathic doctors receive rigorous training in the medical sciences as well as natural therapies, including herbal medicine, acupuncture, nutrition, hydrotherapy, and other modalities.

Although naturopathy has become more mainstream in recent years, it remains a controversial medical approach in some circles.

Critics argue that there is no scientific evidence to support some of the claims made by naturopaths and that some natural therapies can be dangerous if not administered properly.

Despite these criticisms, many people have found relief from chronic health conditions through the use of naturopathic remedies and techniques. As more research is conducted on natural therapies, it is likely that naturopathy will continue to gain acceptance and become more widely used in the healthcare field.

UNDERSTANDING NATUROPATHY TREATMENTS

Naturopathy is a medical system that focuses on natural treatments and therapies to promote overall health and prevent illness. It incorporates a range of non-invasive therapies and treatments that can be used to treat a variety of health conditions.

At the core of naturopathy is the belief that the human body is capable of self-healing. Naturopathic treatments focus on supporting the body's innate healing capacity by providing it with the tools it needs to heal. These tools include nutritional support, herbal medicines, homeopathy, acupuncture, hydrotherapy, and other natural treatments.

Naturopathic treatments are highly individualized and are based on a thorough assessment of the patient's health, including their medical history, current health conditions, symptoms, and lifestyle factors. Naturopathic doctors work closely with their patients to develop a personalized treatment plan that addresses their unique needs and goals.

One of the key principles of naturopathy is the importance of treating the whole person, not just the symptoms of a particular illness or condition. This means that naturopathic treatments may address physical, mental, emotional, and spiritual aspects of a person's health. This holistic approach is designed to support the body's natural healing processes and improve overall well-being.

Some of the most commonly used naturopathic treatments include:

- Herbal Medicine: The use of plants and plant-derived compounds to treat a wide range of health conditions.

- Homeopathy: A holistic healing system that uses highly diluted substances to stimulate the body's natural healing processes.
- Nutritional Therapy: The use of diet, vitamins, and other nutrients to support health and treat illness.
- Acupuncture: A traditional Chinese medicine practice that involves inserting needles into specific points on the body to promote healing and relieve pain.
- Hydrotherapy: The use of water in various forms (such as hot and cold baths, showers, and poultices) to promote healing and alleviate pain.

Other naturopathic treatments may include massage therapy, osteopathy, chiropractic care, and exercise therapy. These treatments are designed to work in harmony with the body's natural healing processes, helping to restore balance and promote optimal health and well-being.

In summary, naturopathy offers a wide range of treatments and therapies that are designed to support the body's natural healing processes. When combined with a healthy lifestyle and regular medical care, naturopathic treatments can be an effective way to promote overall health and well-being.

HOMEOPATHY IN NATUROPATHY

Homeopathy is a form of naturopathic medicine that uses highly diluted substances to stimulate the body's natural healing process. It was developed in the late 18th century by German physician Samuel Hahnemann and has been used widely around the world since then.

Homeopathic remedies are derived from natural substances such as plants, minerals, and animals. The remedies are prepared through a process known as potentization, in which the substance is diluted in water or alcohol and then vigorously shaken or stirred.

The principle behind homeopathy is the "law of similars," which states that a substance that causes certain symptoms in a healthy person can cure those same symptoms in a sick person when administered in highly diluted form. Homeopathic remedies are chosen based on an individual's specific symptoms and overall constitution, rather than a one-size-fits-all approach.

While homeopathy is popular among many people who prefer natural remedies, some critics argue that it lacks scientific evidence and can be dangerous if used to treat certain serious conditions. However, many practitioners and patients attest to the benefits of homeopathy in treating a range of conditions, from allergies and digestive problems to depression and anxiety.

In a homeopathic consultation, the practitioner will first take a detailed medical history and gather information about the patient's overall health and symptoms. The practitioner will then prescribe a specific homeopathic remedy or series of remedies based on the individual's unique case.

Homeopathic remedies are typically taken in the form of small pellets, tablets, or liquid drops. The remedy is usually taken orally and held under the tongue for a brief period before swallowing.

While homeopathy is generally considered safe and well-tolerated, there are some potential side effects and risks to be aware of. Some people may experience temporary worsening of symptoms before experiencing improvement, a phenomenon known as "homeopathic aggravation." Rarely, homeopathic remedies can cause allergic reactions or interact with medications.

Overall, homeopathy provides a natural and individualized approach to healing that can be a valuable addition to a holistic, naturopathic treatment plan. As with any form of alternative medicine, it is important to consult with a qualified practitioner before beginning treatment.

ACUPUNCTURE IN NATUROPATHY

Acupuncture is a traditional Chinese medicine practice that has been used for over 2,000 years. This technique involves the insertion of thin needles into specific points on the body to stimulate energy flow and promote healing. In recent years, acupuncture has become a popular complementary therapy used within naturopathic medicine.

According to traditional Chinese medicine, acupuncture works by balancing the flow of energy (known as Qi) within the body. Blockages or imbalances in Qi are believed to cause illness or pain. By inserting needles in specific points along energy pathways, known as meridians, energy flow can be restored, and health can be improved.

In naturopathic medicine, acupuncture is used to treat a wide range of conditions, from chronic pain and headaches to anxiety and insomnia. It can also be used to promote overall wellness and improve energy levels.

Acupuncture treatment typically begins with an assessment of the patient's overall health and medical history. The practitioner will then identify the specific points on the body to stimulate and insert the needles. Most patients feel little to no discomfort during the procedure, and the needles are left in place for approximately 20-30 minutes.

One of the benefits of acupuncture is that it has very few side effects and is considered safe for most individuals. However, it is important to seek treatment from a qualified acupuncture practitioner who has been properly trained and licensed. In some cases, acupuncture may not be recommended, such as for individuals with bleeding or clotting disorders.

Research has shown that acupuncture can be an effective treatment for a variety of conditions. For example, a study published in the Journal of Pain found that acupuncture was effective in reducing chronic low back pain. Another study published in the Journal of Alternative and Complementary Medicine found that acupuncture improved symptoms of anxiety in patients with chronic obstructive pulmonary disease.

While the use of acupuncture in naturopathic medicine remains somewhat controversial, many individuals have found it to be a helpful complementary therapy. As with any treatment, it is important to speak with a healthcare provider before beginning acupuncture, particularly if you have underlying medical conditions or are taking medications.

TRADITIONAL CHINESE MEDICINE

Traditional Chinese Medicine (TCM) is an ancient healing system that has been used for over 2,500 years in China. It is based on the philosophy of Taoism and the belief that the body's vital energy, or qi, flows through channels known as meridians. When the flow of qi is disrupted or blocked, it can lead to imbalances in the body and cause illness.

TCM is a complex system that includes a range of therapies, such as acupuncture, herbal medicine, cupping, moxibustion, and dietary therapy. Acupuncture, the most well-known form of TCM, involves the insertion of fine needles into specific points along the meridians to restore the flow of qi and promote healing.

Herbal medicine is another important component of TCM. TCM practitioners use a wide variety of herbs, such as ginseng, goji berries, and reishi mushrooms, to treat various ailments. These herbs are often combined in formulas to create a specific effect, such as boosting the immune system, reducing inflammation, or improving digestion.

Cupping and moxibustion are other therapies commonly used in TCM. Cupping involves placing suction cups on the skin to improve circulation and relieve muscle tension, while moxibustion involves burning the herb mugwort near the skin to warm and stimulate specific acupuncture points.

TCM also places a strong emphasis on diet and nutrition. TCM practitioners believe that the foods we eat have a profound impact on our health, and they use dietary therapy to address a wide range of health concerns. For example, a TCM practitioner may recommend certain foods to support digestion, reduce inflammation, or balance hormones.

Overall, TCM is a highly individualized approach to healthcare that takes into account an individual's unique constitution, lifestyle, and environment. By addressing the root causes of illness and promoting balance and harmony in the body, TCM can be an effective way to improve overall health and wellbeing.

AYURVEDA IN NATUROPATHY

Ayurveda is a traditional system of medicine that originated in India over 5000 years ago. It is a holistic approach to health and wellness that focuses on balancing the mind, body, and spirit to promote overall wellness. Ayurveda has become increasingly popular in the West in recent years due to its natural approach to health and wellness.

Ayurvedic medicine operates on the principle that the body is composed of three doshas or energies - Vata, Pitta, and Kapha - which govern its physiological and psychological functions. Maintaining a balance of these doshas is essential for optimal health, and Ayurvedic practitioners use a variety of techniques to help patients restore balance and harmony to their bodies.

One of the primary tools used in Ayurveda is dietary and lifestyle modifications. The Ayurvedic diet stresses the importance of whole, fresh, and nourishing foods tailored to an individual's dosha constitution. This may vary from individual to individual, based on their unique needs and preferences.

Herbal remedies comprise another important aspect of Ayurvedic medicine. Practitioners use a variety of herbs and herbal preparations to address a wide range of health issues. These herbs are typically mixed into a formula tailored to the patient's particular constitution and used in conjunction with other treatment modalities, such as massage and yoga.

Massage is another critical aspect of Ayurvedic medicine. It is regarded as a valuable tool for reducing stress, promoting relaxation, and improving circulation. Ayurvedic massage incorporates techniques such as Abhyanga, an invigorating, warm oil massage that promotes detoxification and relaxation.

Yoga is also an integral part of Ayurvedic medicine. It is a physical and spiritual practice that aims to balance the mind and body through various postures, breathing exercises, and meditation. Ayurvedic practitioners often prescribe a series of yoga asanas tailored to an individual's body type to address specific health concerns.

In summary, Ayurveda is an ancient system of medicine that utilizes natural techniques to promote wellness and health. It provides a holistic approach to health and wellness, emphasizing harmony between the mind, body, and spirit. Alongside other naturopathic treatments, Ayurveda has tremendous potential to transform an individual's health and overall well-being.

NATUROPATHIC NUTRITION

Naturopathic nutrition is the use of diet and nutritional supplements to promote health and treat illness. This approach to nutrition is based on the belief that the body has an innate ability to heal itself and that proper nutrition is essential to supporting this healing process. Naturopathic nutrition practitioners work to identify and address the underlying causes of disease and use specific dietary recommendations and supplements to support the body in achieving optimal health.

The focus of naturopathic nutrition is on the quality of the food we eat, as well as the quantity. Foods that are considered to be nutritious and healing are usually whole, unprocessed, and organic. These foods include fresh fruits and vegetables, whole grains, nuts, seeds, and legumes. Naturopathic practitioners also emphasize the importance of balancing macronutrients (protein, carbohydrates, and fats) and micronutrients (vitamins and minerals) in the diet.

In addition to emphasizing whole, nutrient-dense foods, naturopathic nutrition also promotes the use of dietary supplements to help address specific nutrient deficiencies or to support the body's natural healing processes. These supplements may include vitamins, minerals, amino acids, herbs, and other natural substances.

Naturopathic nutrition practitioners work with clients to create individualized nutrition plans that are tailored to their specific needs and health concerns. They may use a range of tools to assess a client's nutritional status, including physical exams, blood tests, and dietary assessments. From there, they can make recommendations on specific foods, supplements, and dietary practices to support the client's overall health and wellbeing.

Overall, the goal of naturopathic nutrition is to support the body's natural ability to heal itself by providing it with the nutrients it needs to function optimally. By making dietary changes and using specific supplements, naturopathic nutrition can help address a range of health concerns, from digestive issues to chronic disease.

DETOXIFICATION AND CLEANSING

Detoxification and cleansing are two critical aspects of naturopathic medicine. Detoxification is the process of removing harmful toxins and substances from the body, while cleansing involves purifying the blood and organs by removing impurities and waste products. The goal of these methods is to promote optimal health and prevent disease by allowing the body to function at its best.

The Importance of Detoxification and Cleansing

The modern lifestyle exposes us to toxins, pollutants, and chemicals, which can accumulate within our bodies over time, leading to various health problems. The body is designed to deal with a certain amount of toxins; however, when these impurities exceed the body's natural detoxification process, they can lead to many health issues. Some of the common reasons for toxins accumulation include:

- Environmental pollutants
- Unhealthy foods
- Overconsumption of alcohol or drugs
- Chronic stress
- Poor digestion
- Lack of exercise

Detoxification and cleansing can help remove these toxins and impurities, rejuvenating the body and eliminating the risk of many health problems.

The Process of Detoxification and Cleansing

There are several ways a naturopathic practitioner can approach detoxification and cleansing. The body's detoxification process primarily occurs in the liver and kidneys, which filter out and eliminate toxins through urine, sweat, and feces. Some of the methods employed by naturopaths in detoxification and cleansing include:

1. A diet consisting of nutrient-rich foods, including fruits, vegetables, whole grains, lean proteins, healthy fats, and fermented foods.

2. Increased water intake and consumption of herbal teas to help flush out toxins.

3. Fasting or juice fasting to give the digestive system a break and allow the body to focus on detoxifying.

4. Colon cleansing or enemas to remove toxins and waste.

5. Exercise, which can help to reduce chronic inflammation and improve circulation, allowing for more efficient detoxification.

6. Lifestyle changes, including avoiding or minimizing environmental toxins, reducing stress, and adequate sleep.

Benefits of Detoxification and Cleansing

Detoxification and cleansing can have many benefits for your overall health and wellbeing, such as:

- Improved digestion
- Increased energy levels
- Clearer skin
- Better sleep
- Reduced inflammation
- Lowered risk of chronic health problems
- Weight loss

Summary

Detoxification and cleansing are essential components of naturopathic medicine, aimed at helping your body remove toxins and pollutants, promoting overall health and preventing chronic disease. A naturopathic practitioner can help you identify the best approach to detox and cleansing that suits your needs.

HERBAL MEDICINE IN NATUROPATHY

Herbal medicine has been used for centuries as an integral part of traditional medicine systems across the world, and naturopathy is no exception. A naturopathic practitioner may use a wide range of plant-based remedies to help their patients address various medical conditions, whether physical or emotional. In this chapter, we will explore the use of herbal medicine in naturopathy and learn how it provides holistic and effective healthcare.

Herbal medicine encompasses a wide range of natural substances, including plants, flowers, roots, stems, and fruits, which have therapeutic properties. These remedies can be prepared in various forms such as teas, tinctures, extracts, capsules or creams. Naturopathic practitioners use herbal medicine as part of their arsenal to support the body's natural healing ability and promote optimal health outcomes. Herbal medicine is typically customized to an individual's unique medical history, clinical condition, and wellness goals, thereby increasing precision and efficacy.

Some herbal medicines are known for their immune-stimulating properties that allow the body to fight infection or illness. Behind these properties lie potent compounds that can support the immune response and expedite the recovery process. Other herbs exert natural anti-inflammatory properties, such as Curcumin, which can help ease pains and discomforts associated with inflammation. Herbal medicine may also be used to improve the digestive function, enhance mood, reduce stress, anxiety, or depression.

The use of herbal medicine in naturopathy is often combined with other natural healing modalities such as nutrition and lifestyle modifications, for better integration and complementation. For example, a combination of herbal medicine and dietary changes may help to address underlying digestive issues or may help provide the necessary nutrients and vitamins required for proper healing.

As with any medical intervention, herbal medicine must be administered and monitored by a licensed professional, so the specific dosage, duration, and interactions with other herbal medicines or prescription drugs, can be considered. Self-medication without consulting an expert is not advisable and potentially harmful.

In summary, herbal medicine plays a crucial role in the treatment of various medical conditions and symptoms within the natural and holistic approach of naturopathy. Its efficacy, versatility, and individualization make it an excellent candidate for integrative therapies that can work in synergy with the body's innate healing power.

HYDROTHERAPY IN NATUROPATHY

Hydrotherapy, also known as water therapy, is a naturopathic treatment that involves the use of water at different temperatures and pressures to promote healing and relaxation. Hydrotherapy has been used for centuries as a traditional healing method in various parts of the world such as Europe, Asia, and the Middle East.

The practice of hydrotherapy involves the use of water in different forms such as steam, ice, and liquid. The use of water at different temperatures creates various effects on the body, including increased immune activity, increased blood flow, and increased relaxation.

Hydrotherapy can be used to manage different health conditions, including pain relief, promoting immunity, reducing inflammation, and improving blood flow. One of the most common uses of hydrotherapy is pain relief, particularly for individuals with joint pain or muscle aches. The use of heat therapy, such as hot water baths, can help to reduce pain and improve circulation in the affected areas. Cold therapy, such as ice baths or cold compresses, is used to reduce inflammation and promote healing for acute injuries.

Another use of hydrotherapy is to manage stress. The use of water therapy, such as a warm bath or shower, can promote relaxation and reduce stress. The warmth of the water can increase blood flow and help to relax tense muscles, while the sound of water can have a calming effect on the mind.

Hydrotherapy can also be used to improve digestion and promote detoxification. The use of cold water therapy, such as a cold shower or plunge into a cold pool, can stimulate circulation and promote the elimination of toxins from the body. Warm water therapy, such as a sitz bath, can improve digestion and promote bowel movements.

Overall, hydrotherapy is a safe and effective naturopathic treatment that can be used to manage various health conditions. However, it is important to seek the advice of a qualified naturopathic doctor before starting any new treatment.

EXERCISE AND MOVEMENT THERAPY

Exercise is an essential component of any healthy lifestyle, and it plays a critical role in maintaining optimal health and wellbeing. Movement therapy, which involves the use of therapeutic exercises and other movement-based interventions, is a popular approach used in naturopathic medicine to treat and manage a wide range of health conditions.

The goal of exercise and movement therapy is to promote optimal physical health, enhance flexibility and mobility, and improve emotional and mental wellbeing. This chapter will explore the benefits of exercise and movement therapy and how it can be used to improve overall health and wellness.

Benefits of Exercise and Movement Therapy

Exercise has a profound impact on our physical, emotional and mental wellbeing. It helps to improve cardiovascular health and strengthens the immune system, which reduces the risk of chronic diseases, such as heart disease, type 2 diabetes, and obesity. Exercise also enhances cognitive function and reduces the risk of depression and anxiety.

Movement therapy is an effective way to incorporate exercise into a healthy lifestyle, as it is tailored to individual needs and can be used to treat a wide range of health conditions. Movement therapy has been shown to improve balance and mobility, reduce pain, and improve strength and flexibility.

Types of Exercise and Movement Therapy

There are several different types of exercise and movement

therapy used in naturopathic medicine, including:

- Yoga: a form of movement therapy that combines breathing techniques with physical postures to improve flexibility, balance, and mobility.

- Pilates: A system of exercises that strengthen the core muscles and improve balance, coordination, and posture.

- Tai Chi: A form of movement therapy that uses slow, gentle movements to improve balance, reduce stress, and alleviate chronic pain.

- Aerobic Exercise: Activities that increase heart rate and respiratory rate, such as running, cycling or swimming, to improve cardiovascular health and endurance.

- Resistance Training: Exercises that use weights or resistance bands to enhance muscle strength and improve overall fitness.

Conclusion

Exercise and movement therapy are powerful tools that can be used to improve physical, mental, and emotional health. Whether it's through yoga, pilates or aerobic exercise, these approaches have been shown to reduce the risk of chronic disease, improve cardiovascular function, and enhance cognitive function. Naturopathic doctors can work with patients to create a personalized exercise and movement therapy program that meets their individual needs and promotes optimal health and well-being.

INTEGRATIVE MEDICINE
IN NATUROPATHY

Integrative medicine is a holistic approach to healthcare that combines conventional medicine and complementary therapies, including naturopathy. This approach recognizes that no single therapy or approach works for every patient, and that a patient's physical, emotional, and spiritual health should be considered when developing a treatment plan.

Integrative medicine in naturopathy involves the use of multiple therapies to identify and treat the root cause of an illness or disease. Naturopathic doctors work with patients to identify any underlying factors that may be causing health problems, including diet, lifestyle, and emotional well-being.

The use of integrative medicine in naturopathy may involve a range of therapies, including acupuncture, botanical medicine, hydrotherapy, homeopathy, nutrition, and lifestyle counseling. These therapies are used in conjunction with conventional medical treatments, such as prescription medications or surgery, to bring about optimal health outcomes for patients.

One of the key benefits of integrative medicine in naturopathy is the individualized approach to treatment. Rather than relying on a "one-size-fits-all" approach to healthcare, integrative medicine recognizes that each patient is unique and tailors treatment plans to meet their specific needs.

Integrative medicine in naturopathy also places a strong emphasis on preventative care, encouraging patients to take an active role in their own health and well-being. This may involve making changes to diet or lifestyle, incorporating stress-relief techniques, and addressing emotional or psychological factors that may be contributing to poor health.

Incorporating integrative medicine into naturopathic practice requires a strong understanding of both conventional medicine and complementary therapies. Naturopathic doctors who specialize in integrative medicine have undergone additional training in these areas and are able to work collaboratively with other healthcare providers to ensure a comprehensive approach to patient care.

In summary, integrative medicine in naturopathy offers a holistic approach to healthcare that recognizes the interconnected nature of physical, emotional, and spiritual well-being. By combining conventional medicine with complementary therapies, patients can achieve optimal health outcomes while addressing underlying factors that may be contributing to poor health.

STRESS MANAGEMENT AND MIND-BODY THERAPY

In today's fast-paced world, many people experience a high level of stress on a regular basis. Stress is a natural response to challenging situations, but when it becomes chronic or overwhelming, it can negatively impact physical and mental health. Naturopathic medicine offers a variety of stress management techniques, including mind-body therapies, that can help individuals reduce stress and improve overall well-being.

Mind-body therapies are a form of complementary and integrative medicine that emphasize the connection between the mind, body, and spirit. These therapies are designed to improve mental and emotional health by calming the mind and relaxing the body. Examples of mind-body therapies include meditation, deep breathing, yoga, and tai chi.

Meditation is an ancient practice that has been used for thousands of years to calm the mind and promote relaxation. During meditation, individuals focus their attention on a specific object or sound, or simply observe their thoughts and emotions without judgment. Research has shown that regular meditation can reduce stress, anxiety, and depression, as well as lower blood pressure and improve sleep quality.

Deep breathing is another effective stress management technique that can be done anywhere at any time. By breathing slowly and deeply, individuals can activate the parasympathetic nervous system, which helps the body relax and reduces stress. Simple deep breathing exercises can be incorporated into daily life, making it an easy and convenient stress management tool.

Yoga and tai chi are both physical practices that combine movement with deep breathing and relaxation techniques. These practices can help improve flexibility, balance, and strength, while also reducing stress and promoting mental and emotional well-being. They are adaptable to many different fitness levels and can be easily incorporated into a daily routine.

Other naturopathic techniques for stress management include biofeedback, which uses technology to monitor physiological responses to stress and trains individuals to control those responses, and aromatherapy, which uses essential oils to promote relaxation and reduce stress.

In conclusion, chronic stress can have a negative impact on both physical and mental health. Naturopathic medicine provides a variety of mind-body therapies that can help individuals manage stress and improve overall well-being. Incorporating these techniques into a daily routine can promote relaxation and reduce the negative effects of stress on the body and mind.

TREATING CHRONIC CONDITIONS WITH NATUROPATHY

Chronic conditions affect millions of people worldwide, impacting their overall well-being and quality of life. Naturopathy offers a holistic approach to treating chronic conditions, focusing on identifying and addressing root causes rather than just alleviating symptoms.

Naturopathic doctors are trained to work alongside conventional medical professionals to address chronic diseases such as diabetes, arthritis, cardiovascular disease, and autoimmune disorders. They employ a range of natural modalities to help manage chronic conditions, including herbal medicine, acupuncture, and nutritional interventions.

Herbal medicine has been used for centuries to support the body's healing process and address chronic conditions. Herbs such as turmeric, ginger, and ashwagandha have anti-inflammatory properties that can help reduce pain and inflammation associated with chronic conditions. Similarly, adaptogenic herbs such as ginseng and rhodiola can help regulate the body's stress response, which can be beneficial for patients dealing with chronic stress or burnout.

Acupuncture is another popular modality used in supporting the body's natural healing process for many chronic conditions, including pain management, digestive disorders, and mental health concerns. It involves the insertion of thin, sterile needles into specific areas of the body to stimulate healing and promote balance.

Naturopathic doctors may also recommend dietary or lifestyle interventions to help manage chronic conditions, as well as supporting patients with various mind-body techniques. Mind-body therapies such as meditation or yoga may be recommended to help manage stress, which can further worsen underlying chronic conditions if left unaddressed.

Integrating natural therapies and conventional medicine can provide a comprehensive approach to treating chronic conditions, improving overall health outcomes and quality of life for many individuals. Naturopathic approaches are designed to support the body's natural healing process, which can lead to better overall outcomes in the long run.

MANAGING DIGESTIVE DISORDERS WITH NATUROPATHY

Digestive disorders are an increasingly common health issue faced by people all around the world. These disorders can range from minor conditions like acid reflux to serious illnesses like Crohn's disease or ulcerative colitis. Naturopathy offers a variety of approaches to managing digestive disorders, with a focus on identifying and addressing underlying causes rather than simply masking symptoms.

Naturopathic practitioners believe that digestive health is essential for overall well-being. A healthy digestive system promotes the optimal absorption of nutrients and elimination of waste, which in turn supports the immune system and helps to prevent other health problems. Maintaining healthy habits like regular exercise, proper hydration, and a healthy diet can go a long way in promoting digestive health.

When it comes to managing digestive disorders, naturopathy offers a variety of treatment modalities. These may include dietary changes, nutritional supplements, herbal remedies, hydrotherapy, and acupuncture, among others. The specific approach will depend on the individual case, taking into account factors such as the nature and severity of the disorder, the patient's overall health status, and any underlying issues that may be contributing to the problem.

One key area of focus in naturopathic treatment of digestive disorders is identifying and addressing food sensitivities. Many people with chronic digestive problems find relief by eliminating certain problem foods such as gluten, dairy, or processed foods. Nutritional and dietary counseling can help patients to identify problem foods and make appropriate changes to their diet.

Herbal remedies can also play a role in the treatment of digestive disorders. Botanical medicines like peppermint, ginger, or fennel can help to soothe the digestive tract and reduce inflammation. Other herbs like slippery elm or marshmallow root can help to protect the lining of the intestines and promote healing. These remedies are often used alongside dietary changes and other naturopathic modalities.

Digestive disorders can be frustrating and debilitating, but naturopathy offers a holistic approach to managing these conditions. By addressing underlying causes and promoting optimal digestive health, patients can find relief and improve their overall well-being. If you are struggling with a digestive disorder, consider exploring naturopathic approaches to support your healing journey.

NATUROPATHIC APPROACHES TO SKIN HEALTH

The skin is the largest organ in the human body and plays a vital role in protecting the body from external insults, regulating temperature, and eliminating toxins. But for many people, the skin can also be a source of frustration, with conditions like acne, eczema, psoriasis, and rosacea causing discomfort, embarrassment, and even pain.

Naturopathic medicine offers a holistic approach to skin care that goes beyond simply treating symptoms. By addressing the root causes of skin conditions and taking a whole-body approach to health, naturopaths can help their patients achieve clear, healthy, and radiant skin.

Here are some of the ways that naturopathy can support skin health:

1. Addressing nutritional deficiencies: Poor nutrition can manifest in the skin, leading to dryness, flakiness, or even acne. Naturopaths can help identify any nutrient deficiencies and recommend dietary changes or supplements to support healthy skin.

2. Healing the gut: The health of the gut microbiome is closely linked to skin health. Naturopaths can help address digestive issues and dysbiosis in the gut through diet, probiotics, and healing nutrients like glutamine and zinc.

3. Reducing inflammation: Skin conditions like acne and eczema are often caused or exacerbated by inflammation in the body. Naturopaths can recommend anti-inflammatory nutrients like omega-3 fatty acids, curcumin, and quercetin, as well as lifestyle

modifications like stress reduction and exercise.

4. Detoxifying the body: Toxins can accumulate in the body and manifest in the skin, causing rashes, acne, and other issues. Naturopaths can recommend natural detoxification strategies like juice fasts, lymphatic massage, and herbal supplements to help the body eliminate these toxins.

5. Topical treatments: Naturopaths may also recommend topical treatments like herbal creams, essential oils, or clay masks to improve the appearance and health of the skin. These natural remedies can be gentler and less harsh than conventional treatments, which often contain harsh chemicals and synthetic fragrances.

By addressing these underlying causes of skin conditions, naturopaths can help their patients achieve not just clearer, healthier skin, but also greater overall health and vitality.

NATUROPATHIC APPROACHES TO MENTAL HEALTH

Mental health is an integral part of overall well-being, and naturopathy offers various approaches to support mental health. Naturopathic medicine aims to address the root cause of a condition and considers the connection between the mind and body. Integrative approaches may involve dietary changes, supplementation, herbal medicine, acupuncture, and lifestyle modifications. Naturopathic practitioners believe that each person is unique and requires an individualized plan to support their mental health.

Here are some approaches to mental health that naturopathy offers:

1. Diet and Nutrition: A healthy diet and proper nutrition can help improve mood, reduce anxiety, and increase mental focus. Some foods that are beneficial for mental health include fatty fish, nuts, seeds, whole grains, fermented foods, and leafy greens. Naturopathic practitioners may also recommend a diet that is specific to an individual's unique needs.

2. Supplements: Certain supplements can support mental health, including Omega-3 fatty acids, Vitamin D, B-complex vitamins, and magnesium. Naturopathic practitioners may also recommend other supplements that are specific to a person's needs.

3. Herbal Medicine: Herbal medicine can help balance the body's hormones and improve overall mental health. Some herbs that naturopathic practitioners may recommend include ashwagandha, St. John's Wort, passionflower, and chamomile.

4. Acupuncture: Acupuncture can help reduce anxiety and depression by restoring balance to the body's energy channels. Acupuncturists use very thin needles to stimulate specific points on the body, which can restore the flow of energy and promote relaxation.

5. Lifestyle modifications: Naturopathic practitioners may recommend lifestyle modifications that can reduce stress and promote relaxation, such as meditation, yoga, and exercise.

6. Mind-body therapy: Certain mind-body therapies, such as Cognitive Behavioral Therapy (CBT) and Mindfulness-Based Stress Reduction (MBSR) can be beneficial for mental health conditions. Naturopathic practitioners may also recommend other mind-body therapies that are specific to a person's needs.

In conclusion, naturopathic medicine offers many approaches to support mental health. By addressing the root cause of a condition, improving the body's overall balance and offering an individualized plan, naturopathic medicine can help people achieve better mental health and overall wellness.

NATUROPATHY FOR OPTIMAL WELL-BEING

Naturopathy considers the whole person and their overall health when seeking to achieve optimal well-being. By addressing underlying imbalances that may lead to physical and emotional issues, naturopathy provides a holistic approach to health and wellness that emphasizes prevention and addresses the root causes of illness.

One of the primary goals of naturopathy is to support the body's natural healing processes. Naturopathic practitioners use a range of therapies and tools to stimulate and support the body's natural healing abilities, including nutrition, herbal medicine, hydrotherapy, acupuncture, and exercise.

At the core of naturopathic practice is the concept of the healing power of nature, which recognizes that the body has an inherent ability to heal itself. Naturopathy seeks to support and enhance this healing power through natural, non-invasive treatment modalities.

Mental and emotional well-being is also a key aspect of naturopathy. Many naturopathic practitioners recognize that emotional stress can contribute to physical illness, and work with their patients to identify and address underlying emotional imbalances that may be impacting their overall health.

By integrating traditional healing practices with modern scientific research, naturopathy provides a potent combination that can address a wide range of health issues, from chronic conditions like diabetes and heart disease to mental health challenges like anxiety and depression.

Ultimately, naturopathy is about empowering individuals to take control of their health, and to become active participants in their own healing process. By providing a personalized, patient-centered approach to health and wellness care, naturopathy can help individuals achieve optimal well-being, and lead healthier, happier, and more fulfilling lives.